Vagus Stimulation exercises

Conquer Anxiety Naturally: Life-Changing Vagus Nerve Techniques

Mary Dorn

Copyright Page

Copyright © 2025 Mary Dorn

All rights reserved.

No part of this book may be reproduced, stored in a retrieval system, or transmitted in any form or by any means, electronic, mechanical, photocopying, recording, or otherwise, without the prior written permission of the publisher, except for the use of brief quotations in a book review.

Table of Contents

Introduction 6
Chapter 1 10
The Vagus Nerve and Its Role in the Body 10
    Anatomy and Function of the Vagus Nerve 12
    The Vagus Nerve's Connection to the Nervous System 14
    Signs of a Dysfunctional Vagus Nerve 16
Chapter 2 18
The Science Behind Vagus Nerve Stimulation . 18
    How the Vagus Nerve Affects Mental and Physical Health 20
    Scientific Studies on Vagus Nerve Activation .. 24
Chapter 3 33
Breathing Techniques for Vagus Nerve Activation 33
    Diaphragmatic Breathing 35
    Alternate Nostril Breathing 38
    Box Breathing 41
Chapter 4 44
Meditation and Mindfulness for Vagus Nerve Health 44
    Guided Meditation for Relaxation 46
    Mindfulness Practices to Reduce Stress 49
    Body Scanning for Vagus Nerve Stimulation .. 52
Chapter 5 56
Physical Exercises to Stimulate the Vagus Nerve 56
    Gentle Neck and Shoulder Stretches 58

Yoga Poses for Vagus Nerve Activation..........61
Aerobic Exercises for Nervous System Balance. 64

Chapter 6.. 67
Cold Exposure and Vagus Nerve Activation.... 67
Cold Showers and Their Benefits....................69
Ice Baths and Cryotherapy.............................73
Cold Face Immersion for Stress Reduction.... 78

Chapter 7.. 82
Nutrition and Gut Health for Vagus Nerve Function...82
The Gut-Brain Connection............................... 84
Probiotics and Prebiotics for Vagal Tone.........87
Anti-Inflammatory Diet for Nervous System Health...91

Chapter 8.. 100
Sound and Vibration Therapy for the Vagus Nerve.. 100
Humming and Chanting Exercises................102
Singing and Vagus Nerve Stimulation........... 110

Chapter 9.. 121
Emotional Regulation and Vagus Nerve Health... 121
Managing Anxiety Through Vagal Activation.123
The Role of Positive Social Connections...... 128
Journaling and Emotional Expression Techniques... 134

Chapter 10.. 141
Creating a Vagus Nerve Wellness Routine..... 141
Daily Practices for Long-Term Benefits......... 143
Combining Exercises for Maximum

Effectiveness... 151
Tracking Progress and Adjusting Your Routine... 157
Conclusion... **162**
Bonus..**166**
Self Affirmation.. **166**

Introduction

Kamala had always been an ambitious, driven individual. She prided herself on her ability to juggle multiple responsibilities—her career, family, and personal aspirations. But over time, the stress began to take its toll. Sleepless nights, chronic fatigue, and a constant sense of anxiety became her daily companions. No matter how many deep breaths she took or how much she tried to relax, something always felt off. She knew there had to be a deeper, more effective way to regain control over her well-being.

Then, one day, she stumbled upon the concept of the vagus nerve—the body's secret weapon for relaxation, resilience, and healing. She learned that this remarkable nerve, running from the brainstem down through the body, held the key to regulating her stress response, digestion, heart rate, and even mood. More importantly, she discovered that simple, intentional exercises could activate and strengthen her vagus nerve, unlocking a profound sense of calm and vitality.

This book is your guide to harnessing the power of vagus nerve stimulation. Whether you're struggling with anxiety, digestive issues, chronic pain, or simply seeking to enhance your overall well-being, you will find practical, science-backed techniques to support your nervous system. Through targeted exercises, breathwork, mindfulness practices, and lifestyle adjustments, you can unlock the body's innate ability to heal and thrive.

The vagus nerve is not just another piece of the puzzle—it is the missing link to achieving optimal health. By understanding and applying the exercises in this book, you will embark on a transformative journey, one that will leave you feeling more balanced, resilient, and in control of your own well-being.

Your path to a healthier, more energetic life starts today.

Chapter 1

The Vagus Nerve and Its Role in the Body

The vagus nerve is one of the most crucial yet often overlooked components of the human body. As the longest cranial nerve, it plays a significant role in regulating vital functions such as heart rate, digestion, and mood. Understanding the vagus nerve's function and how to optimize its activity can lead to profound improvements in overall health and well-being.

This chapter explores the anatomy and function of the vagus nerve, its connection to the nervous system, and the signs that indicate dysfunction.

Anatomy and Function of the Vagus Nerve

The vagus nerve, also known as the tenth cranial nerve (CN X), originates in the brainstem and extends down through the neck, chest, and abdomen. It branches out to innervate multiple organs, including the heart, lungs, and digestive tract. This extensive network allows it to serve as a communication highway between the brain and various body systems.

Functionally, the vagus nerve is a key player in the parasympathetic nervous system, often referred to as the "rest and digest" system. It helps regulate heart rate, promotes digestion, and facilitates relaxation responses. Additionally, it influences inflammation levels, immune responses, and even emotional well-being by affecting neurotransmitter production.

The Vagus Nerve's Connection to the Nervous System

The nervous system is divided into the central nervous system (CNS) and the peripheral nervous system (PNS). The vagus nerve is a crucial component of the PNS, particularly in its parasympathetic division. While the sympathetic nervous system prepares the body for fight-or-flight responses, the vagus nerve counterbalances this by inducing a state of calm and recovery.

Beyond regulating physiological functions, the vagus nerve plays an essential role in the gut-brain axis. It facilitates communication between the gut microbiome and the brain, influencing mental health and cognitive function. Proper vagal tone, which refers to the nerve's efficiency, is associated with lower stress levels, improved digestion, and enhanced emotional resilience.

Signs of a Dysfunctional Vagus Nerve

When the vagus nerve is not functioning optimally, a range of symptoms can arise, affecting both physical and mental health. Common signs of vagus nerve dysfunction include:

Digestive issues such as bloating, constipation, or acid reflux.

Irregular heart rate or blood pressure fluctuations.

Chronic stress, anxiety, or depression.

Weakened immune function and increased inflammation.

Difficulty swallowing or a hoarse voice.

Low vagal tone is often linked to chronic stress and inflammatory conditions. Fortunately, various techniques, including vagus nerve stimulation exercises, can enhance its function and restore balance to the body.

Understanding the vagus nerve and its impact on overall health is the first step in harnessing its power for healing and wellness. In the following chapters, we will explore effective ways to stimulate and strengthen this vital nerve for improved well-being.

Chapter 2

The Science Behind Vagus Nerve Stimulation

The vagus nerve plays a critical role in maintaining the balance between the body and mind. It acts as a communication superhighway, transmitting signals between the brain and multiple organs, regulating essential functions such as heart rate, digestion, and immune response. Emerging scientific research has illuminated the profound impact vagus nerve stimulation can have on both mental and physical health.

Understanding the science behind this crucial nerve offers a pathway to better well-being and optimized bodily functions.

How the Vagus Nerve Affects Mental and Physical Health

The vagus nerve plays a crucial role in the parasympathetic nervous system, commonly known as the "rest and digest" system. It works to counteract the sympathetic nervous system, which governs the "fight or flight" response. By promoting relaxation and recovery, the vagus nerve helps to maintain homeostasis in the body.

Mental Health Benefits

Reduces Anxiety and Depression: Studies have shown that increased vagal tone correlates with lower levels of stress hormones like cortisol, leading to reduced symptoms of anxiety and depression.

Enhances Emotional Resilience: Stimulation of the vagus nerve can help regulate mood and improve one's ability to cope with emotional stress.

Improves Cognitive Function: Higher vagal activity has been linked to improved memory, focus, and problem-solving skills.

Physical Health Benefits

Lowers Heart Rate and Blood Pressure:
The vagus nerve slows down the heart rate and promotes cardiovascular health, reducing the risk of heart disease.

Aids Digestion: It stimulates the production of digestive enzymes, improving gut health and reducing gastrointestinal disorders like irritable bowel syndrome (IBS).

Boosts Immune Function: A well-functioning vagus nerve enhances the body's ability to fight infections and inflammation.

Regulates Blood Sugar Levels: Vagus nerve stimulation has been associated with improved insulin sensitivity, helping to manage diabetes and metabolic conditions.

Scientific Studies on Vagus Nerve Activation

Over the past few decades, researchers have extensively studied the effects of vagus nerve stimulation (VNS) on human health. Several key findings highlight the potential of VNS as a therapeutic tool.

Neurological and Psychological Research

Depression and Anxiety: Clinical trials have shown that VNS can be an effective treatment for individuals with treatment-resistant depression.

The FDA has approved vagus nerve stimulation therapy for patients who do not respond to conventional antidepressants.

Post-Traumatic Stress Disorder (PTSD): Research indicates that vagal stimulation can help individuals with PTSD by reducing hyperarousal and improving emotional regulation.

Alzheimer's Disease and Cognitive Decline: Scientists have observed that higher vagal tone is associated with better cognitive function, and VNS may have potential in slowing down neurodegenerative diseases.

Cardiovascular Research

Heart Rate Variability (HRV): Studies demonstrate that people with higher HRV, which is directly influenced by the vagus nerve, tend to have lower risks of cardiovascular diseases.

Stroke Recovery: Research has indicated that vagus nerve stimulation can aid stroke patients in regaining motor function more effectively than traditional rehabilitation methods alone.

Gastrointestinal and Inflammatory Studies

Gut-Brain Connection: Scientists have uncovered a strong link between vagal tone and gut microbiome health, influencing digestion, mood, and immune responses.

Chronic Inflammation: A landmark study published in Nature showed that vagus nerve activation could reduce chronic inflammation, making it a promising therapy for autoimmune diseases like rheumatoid arthritis and Crohn's disease.

Benefits of Regular Vagus Nerve Exercises

Engaging in daily practices that stimulate the vagus nerve can lead to long-term health improvements. These exercises promote vagal tone, which enhances overall well-being and resilience against disease.

Psychological and Emotional Benefits

Reduced Stress Levels: Vagus nerve activation lowers cortisol production, leading to a calmer state of mind.

Better Sleep Quality: Stimulation of the vagus nerve has been linked to improved deep sleep cycles, which contribute to mental clarity and physical recovery.

Enhanced Social Connection: Higher vagal tone is associated with better social engagement, making it easier to connect with others and build healthy relationships.

Physical Benefits

Improved Cardiovascular Health: Regular vagus nerve stimulation exercises can help lower blood pressure and improve circulation.

Enhanced Digestive Efficiency: By stimulating the gut-brain axis, these exercises promote healthier digestion and absorption of nutrients.

Boosted Immune System: Increased vagal activity strengthens the body's defense mechanisms against infections and diseases.

Longevity and Overall Well-Being

Anti-Aging Properties: Research suggests that individuals with higher vagal tone tend to have a slower aging process due to reduced inflammation and better cellular function.

Greater Energy Levels: A well-functioning vagus nerve improves mitochondrial efficiency, leading to higher energy production in the body.

Holistic Health Benefits: Engaging in VNS exercises fosters an overall sense of balance, promoting both mental and physical harmony.

The science behind vagus nerve stimulation is both compelling and expansive. Decades of research affirm its crucial role in regulating stress, emotions, heart health, digestion, and immunity. By understanding and harnessing the power of the vagus nerve, individuals can unlock a natural and effective way to enhance their overall well-being.

As we explore further chapters, you will discover practical exercises and techniques to activate this vital nerve, empowering you to take control of your mental and physical health for a more balanced and vibrant life.

Chapter 3

Breathing Techniques for Vagus Nerve Activation

The way we breathe has a profound impact on our nervous system, influencing our stress levels, emotional balance, and overall health. The vagus nerve plays a crucial role in this process, acting as a bridge between the breath and the parasympathetic nervous system—the body's relaxation response.

By practicing specific breathing techniques, we can stimulate the vagus nerve, enhancing its function and promoting a state of calm, improved digestion, and better heart rate variability. This chapter explores three powerful breathing techniques that support vagus nerve activation: diaphragmatic breathing, alternate nostril breathing, and box breathing.

Diaphragmatic Breathing

Also known as belly breathing, diaphragmatic breathing is a fundamental technique for vagus nerve stimulation. This practice involves engaging the diaphragm fully, allowing deeper, more efficient breaths that activate the parasympathetic nervous system.

How to Practice Diaphragmatic Breathing:

Find a comfortable seated or lying position. Position one hand on your chest and the other on your stomach.

Inhale deeply through your nose, directing the breath into your belly so that your abdomen rises while your chest remains still.

Exhale slowly through your mouth, feeling your abdomen deflate as you release the air.

Repeat this process for several minutes, ensuring each inhale and exhale is slow and controlled.

Benefits of Diaphragmatic Breathing:

Lowers heart rate and blood pressure.

Reduces cortisol levels and stress.

Enhances oxygen exchange and lung capacity.

Supports digestion by stimulating the vagus nerve.

Practicing diaphragmatic breathing regularly helps train the body to shift into a parasympathetic state more efficiently, making it a foundational tool for vagus nerve activation.

Alternate Nostril Breathing

Alternate nostril breathing, or Nadi Shodhana, is a yogic technique that balances the nervous system, harmonizes brain activity, and enhances vagal tone. This method helps in clearing the mind, improving focus, and reducing anxiety.

How to Practice Alternate Nostril Breathing:

Sit in a comfortable position with a straight spine and relaxed shoulders.

Use your right thumb to close your right nostril and inhale deeply through the left nostril.

Close your left nostril with your ring finger, release the right nostril, and exhale fully through the right side.

Inhale through the right nostril, then close it and exhale through the left nostril.

Repeat this cycle for several minutes, maintaining a steady rhythm.

Benefits of Alternate Nostril Breathing:

Balances the autonomic nervous system.

Enhances focus and mental clarity.

Reduces stress and promotes relaxation.

Improves lung function and oxygenation.

This technique is particularly beneficial for individuals experiencing high stress or mental fatigue, as it supports a state of inner calm and equilibrium.

Box Breathing

Box breathing, also known as square breathing, is a structured breathing exercise used to regulate stress and improve vagal tone. It is commonly practiced by athletes, military personnel, and individuals seeking mental resilience.

How to Practice Box Breathing:
Sit in a quiet space with an upright posture.
Breathe in deeply through your nose, counting to four.
Hold the breath for four counts.
Exhale gently through your mouth, counting to four.

Hold the breath again for four counts before repeating the cycle.

Continue for 5-10 minutes, maintaining even breath control.

Benefits of Box Breathing:

Reduces stress and anxiety.

Increases focus and mental clarity.

Enhances heart rate variability.

Supports emotional regulation through. vagus nerve stimulation.

Box breathing is an effective tool for anyone seeking to improve their ability to remain calm under pressure and maintain emotional balance.

Breathing is a powerful yet often overlooked tool for enhancing vagus nerve function and promoting overall well-being. Diaphragmatic breathing, alternate nostril breathing, and box breathing each provide unique benefits, but they all share the ability to activate the parasympathetic nervous system, reduce stress, and support a healthier nervous system. By incorporating these techniques into daily routines, individuals can experience a profound shift in their physical and mental health, harnessing the power of the breath to achieve greater balance and resilience.

Chapter 4

Meditation and Mindfulness for Vagus Nerve Health

The vagus nerve plays a crucial role in regulating the body's stress response, promoting relaxation, and supporting overall well-being. One of the most effective ways to enhance vagal tone and stimulate this vital nerve is through meditation and mindfulness. These practices help activate the parasympathetic nervous system, which counterbalances the stress-inducing sympathetic system.

In this chapter, we will explore guided meditation, mindfulness techniques, and body scanning as powerful tools for enhancing vagus nerve function and improving mental and physical health.

Guided Meditation for Relaxation

Guided meditation is a structured approach to meditation where an instructor or recorded voice leads the practitioner through a series of relaxation techniques and visualizations. This method is particularly beneficial for those new to meditation, as it provides a focused and intentional way to engage the mind and body.

Benefits of Guided Meditation for Vagus Nerve Health:

Promotes deep relaxation and reduces stress hormones.

Lowers heart rate and blood pressure.

Enhances vagal tone and parasympathetic activation.

Improves emotional resilience and mental clarity.

How to Practice Guided Meditation:

Find a Quiet Space: Choose a calm environment free from distractions.

Sit or Lie Down Comfortably: Maintain a posture that allows you to relax while keeping your spine aligned.

Use a Guided Recording or App: Many online resources offer guided meditations tailored to relaxation and nervous system balance.

Focus on Your Breath: Follow the narrator's instructions and concentrate on slow, deep breathing.

Engage in Visualization: Imagine a peaceful scene, such as a beach or a forest, to deepen relaxation.

End Gradually: Slowly bring your awareness back to the present moment and stretch gently before resuming daily activities.

Practicing guided meditation for even 10–15 minutes a day can significantly improve vagus nerve function and overall well-being.

Mindfulness Practices to Reduce Stress

Mindfulness involves being completely engaged in the present moment, without any judgment. By cultivating mindfulness, individuals can reduce stress, enhance emotional balance, and stimulate the vagus nerve, thereby improving overall health.

Benefits of Mindfulness for the Vagus Nerve:

Reduces anxiety and depression by increasing vagal tone.

Enhances emotional regulation and self-awareness.

Improves focus and cognitive function.

Supports better digestion and immune response.

Simple Mindfulness Techniques:

Mindful Breathing: Pay attention to each breath, noticing the sensation of air entering and leaving the body.

Body Awareness: Periodically check in with different body parts to release tension.

Mindful Eating: Eat slowly and savor each bite, focusing on textures, flavors, and the act of chewing.

Mindful Walking: Walk slowly and deliberately, paying attention to each step and the sensation of movement.

Gratitude Practice: Take a moment each day to acknowledge and appreciate positive aspects of life.

By integrating mindfulness into daily routines, individuals can effectively stimulate the vagus nerve and foster long-term physical and mental resilience.

Body Scanning for Vagus Nerve Stimulation

Body scanning is a mindfulness technique that involves systematically focusing on different parts of the body, bringing awareness to sensations, and releasing tension. This practice activates the vagus nerve by encouraging relaxation and parasympathetic dominance.

Benefits of Body Scanning:
Reduces physical tension and stress-related discomfort.
Enhances bodily awareness and emotional balance.
Promotes deep relaxation and improves sleep quality.

Strengthens the mind-body connection.

How to Practice Body Scanning:

Lie Down or Sit Comfortably: Choose a relaxed position that allows you to focus without distractions.

Close Your Eyes and Breathe Deeply: Take a few deep breaths to settle into the practice.

Scan from Head to Toe: Bring awareness to each part of the body, starting from the head and moving downward.

Notice Sensations Without Judgment: Observe any areas of tension, warmth, or relaxation without trying to change them.

Release Tension: As you scan each body part, consciously relax any tightness or discomfort.

End with Deep Breathing: Take a few final deep breaths before gently opening your eyes and resuming your day.

Body scanning is particularly effective before bedtime or during high-stress situations, as it helps shift the body into a state of deep relaxation.

Meditation and mindfulness are powerful tools for stimulating the vagus nerve and promoting overall health. Whether through guided meditation, mindfulness techniques, or body scanning, these practices encourage relaxation, reduce stress, and enhance vagal tone. By incorporating these methods into daily life, individuals can experience profound improvements in their mental and physical well-being. Consistency is key, and even small efforts can lead to significant long-term benefits.

Chapter 5

Physical Exercises to Stimulate the Vagus Nerve

The vagus nerve plays a crucial role in regulating many bodily functions, from heart rate and digestion to emotional well-being. While various methods can help stimulate this nerve, physical exercises are among the most effective ways to enhance vagal tone and overall nervous system balance.

In this chapter, we will explore specific exercises designed to activate the vagus nerve, including gentle neck and shoulder stretches, yoga poses, and aerobic exercises.

Gentle Neck and Shoulder Stretches

The vagus nerve runs from the brainstem down through the neck, making gentle movements in this area beneficial for stimulation. By relieving tension in the neck and shoulders, these stretches encourage optimal nerve function and relaxation.

Neck Tilts

Sit or stand with a straight spine.

Slowly tilt your head to the right, bringing your ear toward your shoulder without lifting your shoulder.

Hold for 10-15 seconds, then return to the center.

Repeat on the left side.

Perform 3-5 repetitions per side.

Neck Rotations

Begin with a neutral spine, either seated or standing.

Slowly turn your head to the right, looking over your shoulder.

Hold for 10-15 seconds, then return to the center.

Repeat on the left side.

Perform 3-5 repetitions per side.

Shoulder Rolls

Sit or stand with relaxed shoulders.

Roll your shoulders forward in a circular motion for 10 seconds.

Reverse the motion, rolling them backward for another 10 seconds.

Repeat for 3 sets.

These simple stretches help release muscular tension that could be restricting vagus nerve activity, allowing for improved nervous system function.

Yoga Poses for Vagus Nerve Activation

Yoga is known to enhance vagal tone through breath control, stretching, and relaxation. Specific yoga postures promote vagus nerve stimulation by improving circulation, reducing stress, and encouraging parasympathetic activation.

Cat-Cow Pose (Marjaryasana-Bitilasana)

Begin on all fours in a tabletop position, with your hands and knees on the ground.

Inhale, arch your back, lift your head, and drop your belly (Cow Pose).

Exhale, round your spine, tuck your chin, and draw your navel toward your spine (Cat Pose).

Repeat this flow for 1-2 minutes, coordinating movement with breath.

Bridge Pose (Setu Bandhasana)

Recline on your back with your knees bent and feet positioned hip-width apart.

Place arms alongside your body, palms facing down.

Inhale and lift your hips toward the ceiling while pressing into your feet and shoulders.

Hold for 15-30 seconds, then slowly lower back down.

Repeat 3-5 times.

Legs-Up-the-Wall Pose (Viparita Karani)

Sit sideways against a wall and gently swing your legs up as you lie down.

Rest your arms at your sides, palms facing up.

Close your eyes and focus on slow, deep breathing.

Hold for 5-10 minutes.

These poses help activate the relaxation response, enhance vagal activity, and promote overall nervous system balance.

Aerobic Exercises for Nervous System Balance

Aerobic exercise is another powerful way to stimulate the vagus nerve. Engaging in moderate-intensity cardiovascular activities improves heart rate variability (HRV), which is a key indicator of vagal tone.

Walking

A 30-minute brisk walk can enhance parasympathetic activity.

Walking outdoors, especially in nature, provides additional stress-reducing benefits.

Swimming

Swimming engages the entire body, encourages deep rhythmic breathing, and helps activate the vagus nerve.

Gentle laps or water aerobics for 20-30 minutes can be effective.

Cycling

Riding a bicycle at a moderate pace increases oxygen flow and enhances cardiovascular health.

Aim for 20-45 minutes per session.

Engaging in these activities regularly can improve mood, enhance digestion, and support overall autonomic balance.

Stimulating the vagus nerve through physical exercises is a practical and effective approach to improving nervous system function. Gentle neck and shoulder stretches release tension that may impede vagal activity, yoga poses encourage relaxation and breath control, and aerobic exercises enhance heart rate variability and overall health. By incorporating these exercises into your daily routine, you can support vagus nerve function and experience improved physical and emotional well-being. The key is consistency—small, regular efforts can lead to profound changes over time.

Chapter 6

Cold Exposure and Vagus Nerve Activation

The vagus nerve, a crucial component of the autonomic nervous system, plays a key role in regulating bodily functions such as heart rate, digestion, and stress response. One of the most effective ways to stimulate the vagus nerve is through cold exposure. Cold therapy has been used for centuries to enhance mental and physical resilience, and modern science continues to confirm its benefits for nervous system regulation and overall well-being.

In this chapter, we will explore three powerful cold exposure techniques: cold showers, ice baths, and cold face immersion.

Cold Showers and Their Benefits

Cold showers are one of the simplest and most accessible ways to stimulate the vagus nerve. Unlike traditional warm showers, which promote relaxation and comfort, cold showers create a mild stress response in the body that activates the parasympathetic nervous system. This controlled exposure to cold has numerous physiological and psychological benefits.

How Cold Showers Stimulate the Vagus Nerve

When exposed to cold water, the body experiences an initial shock response, which includes a rapid increase in heart rate and breathing rate. However, after a few moments, the vagus nerve is activated, prompting a shift from the sympathetic (fight-or-flight) response to the parasympathetic (rest-and-digest) state. This transition helps reduce stress, enhance mood, and improve overall nervous system balance.

Benefits of Cold Showers

Reduced Inflammation: Cold water exposure helps lower systemic inflammation, benefiting those with chronic pain and autoimmune conditions.

Enhanced Mood and Mental Clarity: Cold exposure increases the release of endorphins and norepinephrine, which help reduce anxiety and depression.

Improved Circulation: Cold water causes blood vessels to constrict and then dilate, improving blood flow and cardiovascular health.

Strengthened Immune System: Regular cold showers have been linked to increased white blood cell production, leading to enhanced immunity.

How to Take a Vagus Nerve-Stimulating Cold Shower

Start with lukewarm water and gradually lower the temperature.

Focus on deep, controlled breathing to ease the initial shock response.

Expose yourself to the cold water for at least 30 seconds to 2 minutes.

End the shower with cold water to maximize the vagus nerve stimulation.

Ice Baths and Cryotherapy

For those seeking a more intense cold exposure practice, ice baths and cryotherapy offer powerful benefits. These methods involve submerging the body in extremely cold water or exposing it to cold air for a short period. Both techniques have been widely studied for their effects on the nervous system and overall health.

Ice Baths and Their Effects on the Vagus Nerve

Ice baths create a significant drop in skin temperature, which triggers a strong vagal response. As the body adapts, the parasympathetic nervous system is activated, promoting deep relaxation and resilience against stress.

Benefits of Ice Baths

Enhanced Stress Resilience: Regular ice baths train the body to handle stress more effectively, leading to improved mental toughness.

Accelerated Recovery: Athletes and individuals recovering from injuries benefit from the anti-inflammatory and muscle recovery effects of cold immersion.

Improved Sleep Quality: The deep relaxation induced by ice baths helps regulate sleep patterns and improve overall rest.

Boosted Metabolism: Cold exposure increases brown fat activation, which helps regulate body temperature and burn calories efficiently.

How to Safely Take an Ice Bath

Fill a bathtub with cold water and add ice to lower the temperature to around 50-60°F (10-15°C).

Enter slowly, focusing on controlled breathing.

Stay submerged for 2-5 minutes, depending on your tolerance level.

Gradually warm up afterward with gentle movement and warm clothing.

Cryotherapy: An Alternative to Ice Baths

Cryotherapy involves exposing the body to extremely cold air (typically -200°F to -300°F) for a short period in a specialized chamber. This method provides similar benefits to ice baths, including vagus nerve stimulation, reduced inflammation, and enhanced mental clarity. It is often used by athletes, individuals with chronic pain, and those seeking to optimize their nervous system function.

Cold Face Immersion for Stress Reduction

A more targeted method for stimulating the vagus nerve is cold face immersion. This technique involves submerging the face in cold water, which activates the mammalian dive reflex—a physiological response that slows the heart rate and promotes relaxation.

How Cold Face Immersion Stimulates the Vagus Nerve

The mammalian dive reflex is an evolutionary trait found in marine mammals and humans. When the face comes into contact with cold water, the vagus nerve signals the body to lower the heart rate and redirect blood flow to vital organs. This response helps induce a calm and relaxed state, making it an effective method for managing stress and anxiety.

Benefits of Cold Face Immersion

Immediate Stress Relief: Helps calm the nervous system during moments of anxiety or panic.

Reduced Heart Rate: Supports cardiovascular health by promoting vagal tone.

Enhanced Focus and Mental Clarity: Provides a natural way to improve concentration and cognitive function.

Regulation of Blood Pressure: Helps maintain healthy blood pressure levels.

How to Perform Cold Face Immersion

Fill a bowl with cold water and add ice for extra cooling.

Take a deep breath and submerge your face for 10-30 seconds.

Repeat the process 3-5 times, taking breaks between immersions.

Focus on deep breathing to maximize relaxation and vagus nerve activation.

Cold exposure is a powerful, natural tool for stimulating the vagus nerve and enhancing overall well-being. Whether through cold showers, ice baths, or cold face immersion, incorporating these practices into your routine can lead to profound benefits for mental clarity, stress resilience, and physical health. By embracing the discomfort of the cold, you train your nervous system to adapt, recover, and thrive in the face of life's challenges.

In the next chapter, we will explore how nutrition and gut health play a critical role in supporting the vagus nerve and optimizing its function.

Chapter 7

Nutrition and Gut Health for Vagus Nerve Function

In recent years, there has been a surge of interest in understanding how our diet and gut health influence the functioning of the vagus nerve. Once primarily viewed as the body's "communication highway," the vagus nerve has now gained prominence as a key player in our physical and mental well-being. From reducing stress and inflammation to supporting healthy digestion, the vagus nerve's function is intricately linked to our gut health.

With this chapter, we explore the powerful relationship between nutrition, gut health, and vagus nerve function, providing you with actionable insights to optimize your health through mindful dietary choices.

The Gut-Brain Connection

The concept of the gut-brain connection is nothing short of revolutionary. Once thought to be separate systems, the gut and brain are now understood to communicate extensively via the vagus nerve. The gut is commonly known as the "second brain" because of its vast network of neurons, which play a crucial role in regulating numerous bodily functions. processes, including digestion, immunity, and even mood regulation.

The vagus nerve, one of the longest cranial nerves, connects the brain to the gut, creating a bidirectional communication system. Signals travel from the gut to the brain, alerting it to changes in digestive processes, while also conveying messages from the brain to the gut that can influence gastrointestinal motility, enzyme secretion, and gut barrier function.

This ongoing conversation between the brain and gut is critical for overall health. For example, when the gut is under stress (due to poor diet, inflammation, or microbial imbalances), it can send distress signals to the brain, leading to anxiety, depression, and cognitive impairment.

Similarly, mental stress can alter gut function by disrupting the balance of gut microbes, leading to digestive issues, immune dysfunction, and even chronic diseases.

For this reason, maintaining a healthy gut is not just beneficial for digestion but is also essential for mental clarity, emotional balance, and overall nervous system health. Understanding the gut-brain axis and nurturing it through dietary and lifestyle practices can greatly enhance vagus nerve function, boosting both physical and mental resilience.

Probiotics and Prebiotics for Vagal Tone

Probiotics and prebiotics are two important dietary components that play a significant role in shaping the gut microbiome—the ecosystem of microorganisms living in the digestive tract. These microorganisms are critical for regulating the immune system, aiding digestion, and even supporting the function of the vagus nerve.

Probiotics, also known as "beneficial bacteria," are live microorganisms that support overall health, especially gut function, when consumed in sufficient quantities.

They are commonly found in fermented foods such as yogurt, kefir, sauerkraut, kimchi, and kombucha. These foods help maintain a healthy microbial balance in the gut by introducing beneficial bacteria that support digestion, reduce inflammation, and even enhance vagus nerve activity.

Regular consumption of probiotics can enhance vagal tone by promoting the growth of specific beneficial bacteria that are known to reduce gut permeability and modulate the immune response.

This, in turn, leads to a reduction in gut-derived inflammation, which has been linked to poor vagal function and various chronic diseases, including autoimmune disorders and neurological conditions.

Prebiotics, on the other hand, are types of fiber that the human body cannot digest but which serve as food for beneficial gut bacteria. Prebiotics are found in many plant-based foods, including garlic, onions, leeks, asparagus, bananas, and whole grains. These fibrous foods help promote the growth and activity of probiotics in the gut, creating an optimal environment for the gut microbiome and, consequently, enhancing vagal function.

When the gut microbiome is in balance, it facilitates optimal communication between the gut and brain, strengthening the vagus nerve's ability to regulate physiological processes such as inflammation, stress response, and digestion. The connection between probiotics, prebiotics, and the vagus nerve suggests that nurturing the gut microbiome through proper nutrition can significantly enhance the function of this vital nerve.

Anti-Inflammatory Diet for Nervous System Health

Inflammation is one of the body's natural responses to injury or infection, but when it becomes chronic, it can lead to a wide range of health problems. Chronic inflammation is now considered one of the primary contributors to many neurological and gastrointestinal disorders, including depression, anxiety, autoimmune diseases, and neurodegenerative conditions.

The vagus nerve plays a crucial role in regulating the body's inflammatory response through the inflammatory reflex. This is a process by which the vagus nerve sends signals to the brain to reduce the production of pro-inflammatory molecules, thereby helping to maintain immune system balance. When vagus nerve function is optimal, it helps keep inflammation in check. However, when the vagus nerve is underactive, the body's inflammatory response can become dysregulated, leading to chronic low-grade inflammation, which can contribute to the development of numerous health issues.

One of the most effective ways to support vagus nerve function and reduce chronic inflammation is through a balanced, anti-inflammatory diet. Such a diet focuses on nutrient-dense foods that help calm inflammation and nourish the body, providing the necessary building blocks for optimal nerve function.

Foods that are rich in omega-3 fatty acids, such as fatty fish (salmon, mackerel, sardines), flaxseeds, chia seeds, and walnuts, have been shown to reduce inflammation in the body and support the vagus nerve. Omega-3s help regulate the production of pro-inflammatory cytokines, reducing the risk of chronic inflammation and promoting healthy nervous system function.

Antioxidant-rich foods such as berries, dark leafy greens, and cruciferous vegetables (like broccoli and Brussels sprouts) are also essential for reducing oxidative stress and inflammation.

These foods contain compounds that neutralize harmful free radicals, which are associated with both inflammation and aging-related damage to the nervous system.

Polyphenols, found in foods such as turmeric, green tea, dark chocolate, and olives, also have potent anti-inflammatory effects. One of the most well-studied polyphenols, curcumin, found in turmeric, has been shown to enhance vagus nerve activity by reducing inflammation and promoting healthy brain function.

A key focus of an anti-inflammatory diet is the reduction of processed foods, refined sugars, and trans fats, which are known to contribute to chronic inflammation. By removing or limiting these inflammatory triggers from the diet, you can help reduce the burden of inflammation on the body and support a more balanced immune system, improving the function of the vagus nerve.

By focusing on anti-inflammatory foods, you can actively reduce the body's inflammation levels, boost the function of your vagus nerve, and optimize your overall health. Coupled with regular exercise, stress management, and other vagus nerve-stimulating practices, a diet rich in anti-inflammatory foods can contribute to a stronger, more resilient nervous system.

In this chapter, we've explored the critical link between gut health, nutrition, and vagus nerve function. By understanding the gut-brain connection and recognizing the powerful impact of probiotics, prebiotics, and anti-inflammatory diets, you now have the tools to foster better vagal tone and, in turn, enhance your physical and mental well-being.

Nurturing your gut health with the right nutrition is a holistic and practical way to optimize your vagus nerve's function, paving the way for reduced inflammation, better digestion, improved emotional regulation, and a more resilient nervous system.

Start incorporating these dietary changes today, and you'll begin to experience the profound benefits that come with a healthy, active vagus nerve. The connection between what we eat, how we feel, and the performance of our body's vital systems has never been more clear, and it's time to make that connection work for you.

Chapter 8

Sound and Vibration Therapy for the Vagus Nerve

Sound and vibration have long been used for healing purposes across cultures and civilizations. From the hum of Tibetan singing bowls to the chants of ancient monks, the therapeutic power of sound has been recognized for centuries. Today, we're uncovering the connection between sound therapy and the vagus nerve—a powerful communication pathway that influences everything from our stress levels to our emotional regulation.

As science catches up with ancient wisdom, we now understand that sound and vibration not only soothe the mind but also play a crucial role in enhancing vagus nerve function. In this chapter, we delve into the fascinating world of sound and vibration therapy, exploring how these practices can stimulate the vagus nerve, improve health, and foster a greater sense of calm.

Humming and Chanting Exercises

Humming and chanting exercises are among the simplest and most effective ways to stimulate the vagus nerve. The unique combination of sound and vibration created by these practices provides a direct and profound impact on the body's nervous system, encouraging the parasympathetic nervous system to engage, which helps calm the body and mind. Humming, in particular, produces a low-frequency vibration that resonates through the head, neck, and chest, directly stimulating the vagus nerve.

This process is often referred to as "vagal toning," as it helps improve the tone and responsiveness of the vagus nerve, allowing it to better regulate vital functions such as heart rate, digestion, and stress levels.

Humming as a Vagus Nerve Stimulator

The act of humming involves gentle vibrations in the throat, which have been shown to positively influence the vagus nerve. When we hum, air moves through the vocal cords, creating a vibration that resonates in the nasal passages and the upper respiratory tract.

This resonance helps activate the vagus nerve, particularly in the areas it innervates, including the larynx, diaphragm, and heart. As a result, humming can help reduce stress, lower blood pressure, and regulate heart rate, offering a simple and natural tool for fostering relaxation.

In addition to its physical benefits, humming can also have a profound effect on mental well-being. The vibration and resonance created during humming can lead to a state of deep calm and relaxation. Research has shown that this practice may lower levels of cortisol, the hormone associated with stress, and increase levels of oxytocin, a hormone linked to feelings of trust and social bonding. These physiological changes make humming an effective tool for combating anxiety and depression, improving emotional regulation, and fostering a sense of inner peace.

Chanting and Mantras for Vagal Stimulation

Chanting, particularly with the repetition of mantras or sacred sounds, offers similar benefits to humming while introducing a meditative element to the practice. Chanting has been used in various cultures, particularly in Hinduism and Buddhism, as a means of focusing the mind and achieving spiritual elevation. Modern science now recognizes that these practices also have a profound impact on the body's nervous system.

When chanting, the continuous repetition of a specific sound or mantra not only generates a sound vibration but also encourages mindful breathing, both of which stimulate the vagus nerve. The rhythmic pattern of chanting and the deep, steady breathing involved in the practice trigger the parasympathetic nervous system, inducing a relaxation response that can help reduce stress and anxiety, improve mood, and lower heart rate and blood pressure.

The ancient yogic mantra "Om," for example, is often chanted to create a deep sense of tranquility and connection to the present moment. The resonance produced by the chanting of "Om" vibrates through the chest and head, stimulating the vagus nerve, improving vagal tone, and supporting both physical and mental well-being.

How to Practice Humming and Chanting

To begin using humming and chanting for vagus nerve stimulation, find a quiet space where you can relax without distractions. Sit in a relaxed position with your spine straight, close your eyes, and take a few deep breaths to ground yourself.

Then, begin humming gently. Focus on the vibrations in your throat and chest as you hum, allowing the sound to resonate deeply. You may find that as you hum, your breath slows, your body relaxes, and your mind calms.

For chanting, select a mantra or phrase that resonates with you. It can be a traditional mantra, a personal affirmation, or simply a word that brings you peace. Begin chanting slowly and steadily, aligning your breath with the rhythm of the chant. You may repeat the mantra for several minutes, allowing the vibrations and sound to wash over you.

Singing and Vagus Nerve Stimulation

Singing, much like humming and chanting, is another powerful tool for stimulating the vagus nerve. When we sing, especially at a slow, controlled pace, we engage in diaphragmatic breathing, a technique that has long been known to activate the parasympathetic nervous system. The deep, full breaths required in singing help reduce stress levels, regulate the heart rate, and improve lung function.

The Connection Between Singing and Vagal Tone

Singing not only promotes healthy breathing but also helps improve vagal tone by increasing the variability of heart rate. This variability—known as heart rate variability (HRV)—is a key indicator of the health of the vagus nerve. High HRV is associated with greater resilience to stress and better autonomic nervous system balance, both of which are influenced by the vagus nerve. Singing, with its rhythm, breath control, and vocalization, helps increase HRV, thereby supporting vagus nerve function.

The physical act of singing can also be particularly beneficial for individuals experiencing stress or anxiety. Singing has been shown to release endorphins, the body's natural "feel-good" hormones, and to increase the production of oxytocin, which promotes relaxation and social bonding. These chemical changes, coupled with the deep breathing involved in singing, make it an excellent practice for emotional and physical healing.

The Therapeutic Power of Group Singing

Group singing, such as in choirs or communal singing circles, can have even more profound effects on vagus nerve stimulation. The shared experience of singing together can foster a sense of community, belonging, and connection. The act of synchronizing breath and voice with others creates a collective resonance that can deeply enhance vagal tone. This shared experience often results in a powerful emotional release, helping to improve mental well-being and decrease feelings of isolation or loneliness.

How to Incorporate Singing into Your Routine

To incorporate singing into your routine, start by choosing songs that you enjoy and feel comfortable singing. Begin by singing along to your favorite tunes, paying attention to your breath and vocal control. As you sing, focus on taking deep, diaphragmatic breaths, allowing your lungs to expand fully with each inhalation. With time, singing can become a joyful and relaxing ritual that enhances your vagus nerve function, improves your mood, and supports overall well-being.

Sound Frequencies and Healing Vibrations

Beyond humming, chanting, and singing, sound frequencies and vibrations also offer a powerful means of stimulating the vagus nerve and supporting overall health. Sound therapy, using specific frequencies or vibrations, has been used for centuries in various healing practices. Modern science has begun to explore how different frequencies can influence the nervous system, including the vagus nerve, and provide therapeutic benefits for both physical and emotional health.

Binaural Beats and Vagus Nerve Stimulation

One of the most well-known sound therapy techniques is the use of binaural beats. Binaural beats involve playing two slightly different frequencies in each ear, which the brain perceives as a single, rhythmic beat. Research has shown that listening to binaural beats can have a profound effect on the brain, promoting relaxation, improving focus, and even enhancing vagal tone.

The frequency range most associated with vagus nerve stimulation is in the alpha and theta ranges (8-12 Hz and 4-8 Hz, respectively). Listening to binaural beats in these frequencies can help increase heart rate variability, reduce stress, and promote overall relaxation. The brain's response to these frequencies can help engage the parasympathetic nervous system and enhance the body's natural ability to self-regulate.

Sound Therapy Instruments

In addition to binaural beats, various sound therapy instruments are used for vagus nerve stimulation. These include singing bowls, gongs, tuning forks, and crystal bowls. These instruments produce a range of frequencies and vibrations that penetrate the body's tissues, helping to balance the autonomic nervous system, reduce stress, and promote healing.

How to Use Sound Frequencies in Your Practice

To incorporate sound frequencies into your wellness routine, consider listening to binaural beats or attending sound healing sessions. Many apps and platforms now offer audio tracks designed specifically to target vagus nerve stimulation and enhance relaxation. Whether you're listening to these tracks during meditation, before sleep, or while engaging in light stretching, sound therapy can provide a potent boost to your vagus nerve function and overall health.

In this chapter, we've explored the power of sound and vibration therapy for stimulating the vagus nerve. Whether through humming, chanting, singing, or sound frequencies, these practices offer a unique and accessible way to enhance vagal tone, improve mental and emotional health, and support overall well-being. By integrating these practices into your daily routine, you can harness the therapeutic power of sound to reduce stress, regulate your nervous system, and foster a deeper sense of relaxation and balance. The relationship between sound, vibration, and the vagus nerve is a fascinating and powerful one, and it holds the key to unlocking a wealth of benefits for both the body and mind.

Chapter 9

Emotional Regulation and Vagus Nerve Health

Managing emotions effectively is essential for mental health and overall well-being. The ability to effectively manage and respond to emotional experiences can significantly impact our daily lives, influencing everything from stress levels to interpersonal relationships. One of the key players in emotional regulation is the vagus nerve, a major nerve in the autonomic nervous system that acts as a vital link between the brain as well as multiple organs, such as the heart, lungs, and digestive system.

In this chapter, we explore the profound connection between the vagus nerve and emotional regulation, focusing on how vagal activation can improve mental health, reduce anxiety, and foster healthier emotional responses. Through various techniques such as managing anxiety, fostering positive social connections, and incorporating journaling and emotional expression practices, we can enhance vagus nerve health and cultivate a more balanced, resilient emotional state.

Managing Anxiety Through Vagal Activation

Anxiety is a common and debilitating emotional experience that affects millions of people worldwide. Characterized by excessive worry, nervousness, and a constant sense of unease, anxiety can take a significant toll on both mental and physical health. However, recent research has highlighted the important role that the vagus nerve plays in modulating anxiety and stress responses. By activating the vagus nerve, we can enhance our body's ability to regulate the autonomic nervous system, leading to a reduction in anxiety symptoms and promoting overall emotional well-being.

The Science of Vagal Activation for Anxiety

The vagus nerve plays a crucial role in the parasympathetic nervous system, which controls the body's "rest and digest" functions. When activated, the vagus nerve triggers the release of calming neurotransmitters such as acetylcholine, which help slow down the heart rate, lower blood pressure, and promote relaxation. This activation counteracts the "fight or flight" response of the sympathetic nervous system, which is often triggered during anxiety-inducing situations.

By stimulating the vagus nerve, we can shift our body from a state of heightened stress to one of calm and balance.

Research has shown that practices such as deep breathing, meditation, and other forms of vagus nerve stimulation can help increase vagal tone—the ability of the vagus nerve to regulate bodily functions effectively. A higher vagal tone is associated with better emotional regulation, greater resilience to stress, and a reduced risk of anxiety and depression. Conversely, a low vagal tone can make it more difficult to manage stress and anxiety, leading to a higher likelihood of experiencing negative emotional states.

Techniques for Activating the Vagus Nerve to Reduce Anxiety

There are several practical methods for activating the vagus nerve and managing anxiety. One of the most effective techniques is deep diaphragmatic breathing, which involves slow, deep breaths that engage the diaphragm and stimulate the vagus nerve. As you inhale deeply and exhale slowly, you trigger the parasympathetic nervous system, promoting relaxation and reducing feelings of anxiety.

Another technique for vagal activation is cold exposure, such as cold showers or splashing cold water on your face. The sudden shock of cold stimulates the vagus nerve and helps regulate the body's stress response. Other practices, such as chanting, humming, and even singing, have also been shown to activate the vagus nerve and promote emotional calm.

By regularly practicing these techniques, you can strengthen your vagus nerve and improve your ability to manage anxiety. Whether through breathing exercises, cold exposure, or sound therapy, activating the vagus nerve offers a powerful and natural way to combat anxiety and enhance emotional well-being.

The Role of Positive Social Connections

Human beings are inherently social creatures, and our emotional well-being is closely linked to the quality of our social connections. Research has shown that positive social relationships play a crucial role in regulating emotions, reducing stress, and promoting overall health. But what does this have to do with the vagus nerve?

The vagus nerve is not only involved in the regulation of physiological functions but also plays an important role in emotional regulation during social interactions.

In fact, the vagus nerve is often referred to as the "social nerve" because of its involvement in the physiological processes that facilitate social bonding and connection. When we interact with others in a positive and supportive way, the vagus nerve helps regulate our emotional responses, allowing us to feel safe, calm, and connected.

The Vagus Nerve and the Social Engagement System

One of the primary functions of the vagus nerve is its involvement in the "social engagement system," a term coined by Dr. Stephen Porges, a researcher and clinician in the field of neurobiology.

According to Porges' Polyvagal Theory, the vagus nerve helps regulate our physiological responses during social interactions, including facial expressions, vocalizations, and eye contact. These cues are essential for building trust, empathy, and emotional connection with others.

When we experience positive social interactions, our vagus nerve is activated, leading to a reduction in stress hormones such as cortisol and an increase in feelings of safety and well-being. This social engagement response not only helps us regulate our emotions but also supports our physical health, as it promotes relaxation, reduces inflammation, and enhances immune function.

Conversely, negative social interactions, such as conflict, rejection, or isolation, can lead to a reduction in vagal tone, which can make it more difficult to manage emotions and respond to stress. This is why building and maintaining positive social relationships is so important for mental health. By fostering meaningful connections with others, we can enhance our vagal tone and improve our ability to regulate emotions effectively.

Nurturing Positive Social Connections

To nurture positive social connections and support vagus nerve health, consider the following practices:

Engage in meaningful conversations: Deep, authentic conversations help create a sense of connection and trust, both of which activate the vagus nerve and promote emotional regulation.

Practice active listening: By truly listening to others, we enhance the quality of our interactions and create a sense of empathy and understanding, fostering positive relationships.

Spend time with loved ones: Regularly spending time with friends, family, or other supportive individuals helps create a sense of belonging and reduces feelings of loneliness or isolation.

Engage in social activities: Participating in group activities, such as community events or group exercise, can help strengthen social bonds and improve emotional well-being.

By prioritizing positive social connections, we can strengthen our vagus nerve, improve our emotional regulation, and enhance our overall mental and physical health.

Journaling and Emotional Expression Techniques

Journaling and emotional expression are powerful tools for regulating emotions, especially when dealing with stress, anxiety, or difficult feelings. Writing allows us to process our thoughts, explore our emotions, and gain clarity about our experiences. This practice not only helps us understand ourselves better but also supports the health of our vagus nerve.

The Therapeutic Benefits of Journaling

Journaling has long been recognized as a therapeutic practice for emotional well-being. Writing about our experiences allows us to release pent-up emotions, reduce stress, and gain perspective on our challenges. In fact, research has shown that expressive writing can help lower cortisol levels, the stress hormone, and improve overall emotional health. When we write about our thoughts and feelings, we engage in a form of emotional expression that can help us process difficult emotions and release them from our minds and bodies.

Journaling can also enhance vagal tone by promoting emotional regulation. By regularly reflecting on our emotions and experiences, we become more attuned to our inner states and develop better strategies for managing stress and anxiety. This self-awareness is crucial for improving vagus nerve function, as it helps us identify triggers that may activate the sympathetic nervous system and learn how to counteract them with calming techniques.

Expressive Writing for Emotional Release

In addition to traditional journaling, expressive writing techniques can be particularly effective for emotional release. Expressive writing involves writing freely and without judgment about emotions, experiences, or memories, allowing the writer to explore their deepest feelings and gain insight into their emotional responses. This type of writing can help process trauma, reduce emotional reactivity, and foster a sense of emotional release and catharsis.

How to Practice Journaling and Emotional Expression

To incorporate journaling into your emotional regulation routine, start by setting aside time each day or week to write about your thoughts and feelings. You can write in a traditional journal, create a digital log, or even engage in free-form expressive writing. Focus on expressing your emotions honestly and without judgment, allowing the words to flow naturally.

Consider using prompts to guide your journaling practice. Some examples include:

"What emotions am I experiencing at this moment, and what is causing them?"

"What stressors am I currently facing, and how can I cope with them?"

"What brings me a sense of peace, and how can I invite more of it into my daily life?"

By using journaling and emotional expression techniques, you can enhance your emotional regulation, reduce stress, and support the health of your vagus nerve.

In this chapter, we have explored the powerful connection between emotional regulation and vagus nerve health. Through techniques such as managing anxiety through vagal activation, fostering positive social connections, and engaging in journaling and emotional expression practices, we can enhance vagal tone and improve our ability to regulate emotions effectively. The vagus nerve plays a central role in our emotional well-being, and by nurturing its health, we can foster a greater sense of calm, resilience, and balance in our lives.

Chapter 10

Creating a Vagus Nerve Wellness Routine

In the quest for a balanced, healthy, and resilient body and mind, the vagus nerve holds a central position. Known as the "wandering nerve" due to its far-reaching pathways through the body, it plays a pivotal role in regulating numerous systems, from heart rate to digestion, and from immune function to emotional regulation. Strengthening the vagus nerve through a comprehensive wellness routine can lead to profound improvements in both physical and mental well-being.

Creating a well-rounded, personalized vagus nerve wellness routine is essential for achieving long-term health benefits, fostering resilience against stress, and promoting a balanced autonomic nervous system. This chapter provides a practical guide for developing such a routine, which integrates daily practices, combines exercises for maximum effectiveness, and emphasizes the importance of tracking progress. With consistent effort, a thoughtfully designed vagus nerve wellness routine can transform your health, enhance your emotional regulation, and improve your overall quality of life.

Daily Practices for Long-Term Benefits

Establishing a daily routine centered around vagus nerve health is a crucial step toward reaping the long-term benefits of vagal tone improvement. The key is consistency. By engaging in practices that activate and stimulate the vagus nerve every day, you can gradually build up its efficiency and effectiveness in regulating bodily functions. Over time, these habits will help you manage stress more effectively, enhance emotional resilience, and promote overall well-being.

Breathing Techniques

One of the simplest and most effective ways to engage the vagus nerve daily is through controlled breathing. Deep diaphragmatic breathing, where you focus on slow, deep inhales and exhales, directly stimulates the vagus nerve. By slowing the breath and lengthening each inhale and exhale, you engage the parasympathetic nervous system, signaling the body to relax. As a result, your heart rate slows, blood pressure stabilizes, and feelings of anxiety are reduced. To gain the full benefits of this practice, consider dedicating five to ten minutes each day to deep breathing exercises.

Techniques such as box breathing, alternate nostril breathing, or abdominal breathing are excellent ways to activate the vagus nerve.

Meditation and Mindfulness

Meditation and mindfulness exercises serve as potent tools for regulating the vagus nerve and achieving mental clarity. Mindfulness practices—such as focusing on the present moment and cultivating an awareness of your thoughts and feelings without judgment—engage the parasympathetic nervous system.

Mindful practices such as guided meditation, body scanning, and progressive muscle relaxation can help reduce stress and activate the vagus nerve by fostering deep relaxation. By dedicating time each day to mindful meditation, you create a mental space where your vagus nerve can thrive, improving emotional regulation, and decreasing anxiety.

Cold Exposure

Cold exposure, such as cold showers or splashing cold water on your face, is another effective practice for stimulating the vagus nerve daily. The sudden exposure to cold stimulates the vagus nerve, promoting a parasympathetic response and reducing feelings of stress. Starting your day with a cold shower or incorporating cold water immersion into your routine can help increase vagal tone, boost energy levels, and enhance resilience to stress. For many people, a brief burst of cold exposure in the morning or before a stressful event can serve as an effective reset, helping to ground and center the nervous system.

Gentle Physical Activity

Incorporating gentle forms of physical activity into your daily routine is essential for overall health and vagus nerve stimulation. Activities such as yoga, Tai Chi, and light stretching not only activate the vagus nerve but also promote flexibility, balance, and relaxation. Consider integrating simple stretches into your morning routine or attending a weekly yoga class that focuses on deep breathing and relaxation. Gentle physical exercise is not only good for the body but also supports the body's parasympathetic functions, making it a perfect addition to any wellness routine.

Social Connections and Positive Interactions

The vagus nerve is heavily involved in our social interactions, and building meaningful, positive social connections is essential for long-term wellness. Engaging in daily conversations, spending time with friends or family, or participating in community activities stimulates the vagus nerve and promotes feelings of safety and relaxation. The positive emotional feedback from social interactions leads to the release of neurochemicals that activate the parasympathetic nervous system, reducing stress and fostering emotional balance.

Make it a priority to engage with others in meaningful ways each day to enhance vagal tone and emotional well-being.

Combining Exercises for Maximum Effectiveness

While each of the practices outlined in the previous section has its own set of benefits, combining them into a holistic, integrated routine can enhance their effectiveness and yield greater results. It is essential to approach vagus nerve activation from multiple angles to create a well-rounded, balanced wellness routine. Combining practices not only strengthens the vagus nerve but also enhances the body's overall ability to regulate the autonomic nervous system.

Create a Balanced Morning Routine

Start your day with a series of exercises that activate the vagus nerve and promote calmness. Begin with a session of diaphragmatic breathing to center your body and mind, followed by a short meditation to focus and reduce stress. Then, integrate gentle neck and shoulder stretches or yoga poses to increase circulation and relieve tension. A brief cold exposure, such as a splash of cold water to the face or a quick cold shower, can help refresh and invigorate the body while stimulating the vagus nerve.

A morning routine like this prepares you for the day ahead, setting a tone of calm and balance.

Integrating Movement with Breathwork

Physical exercise, when combined with focused breathwork, can be incredibly powerful for vagus nerve stimulation. For example, incorporating deep breathing into your daily walk or light jog can enhance the calming effects of exercise, leading to better overall vagal tone. Try focusing on breathing deeply and consciously as you move, whether you're walking, cycling, or performing light resistance training.

This combination of movement and breath helps maintain a balanced autonomic nervous system, improving heart rate variability and overall resilience to stress.

Use Music and Sound to Enhance Your Routine

Sound-based exercises, such as humming, chanting, or singing, have been shown to activate the vagus nerve and improve emotional regulation. You can combine this practice with other exercises to enhance your routine further. For example, try humming softly during your meditation or singing a favorite song during your walk.

The vibrations created during vocalization stimulate the vagus nerve and promote relaxation. This combination of breath, sound, and movement creates a dynamic, holistic practice for vagus nerve wellness.

End Your Day with Relaxing Rituals

Ending your day with relaxation techniques ensures that your body and mind remain balanced. After a busy day, engage in gentle stretching or restorative yoga poses to release any built-up tension. Follow this with a brief meditation or mindfulness practice, allowing your thoughts to settle.

Journaling can also be an effective way to process your day and release lingering emotions. Ending your day with calming activities prepares you for restful sleep, ensuring that your vagus nerve is operating at its optimal level.

Tracking Progress and Adjusting Your Routine

Like any wellness journey, it is important to track your progress and adjust your routine as needed. The body's response to vagus nerve stimulation can vary from person to person, and what works for one individual may not work for another. Monitoring your progress and making adjustments ensures that your routine is personalized, effective, and sustainable over time.

Keep a Wellness Journal

Monitoring your progress can be as easy as maintaining a journal. Record your daily practices, including the techniques you are using, how long you engage in each activity, and any changes you notice in your physical or emotional state. Journaling your experience helps you stay accountable and gives you insight into what works best for you. Over time, you will be able to identify patterns, strengths, and areas for improvement.

Assess Your Emotional and Physical Responses

As you engage in your routine, take note of any shifts in your emotional and physical state. Are you feeling less anxious or more grounded? Are you experiencing better sleep or improved digestion? Tracking these changes can help you determine the effectiveness of your routine and highlight areas that may need more attention. For example, if you find that you're struggling with anxiety despite practicing vagus nerve exercises, you may want to adjust the intensity or frequency of your techniques, or try adding new ones to your routine.

Make Adjustments as Needed

Your wellness routine should evolve as your needs change. If you notice that certain techniques are no longer as effective or that new challenges have emerged, don't hesitate to adjust your practices. You might find that incorporating more breathwork or adding a new physical exercise to your routine helps address a new stressor. Continuously fine-tuning your routine based on your body's feedback is essential for maintaining progress and achieving long-term benefits.

Creating a vagus nerve wellness routine is an ongoing journey that requires dedication, self-awareness, and consistency. By integrating daily practices such as breathwork, meditation, cold exposure, physical activity, and social connections, you can improve vagal tone and enhance emotional regulation. Combining exercises for maximum effectiveness and tracking your progress ensures that your routine remains personalized and adaptable over time. With patience and persistence, a well-crafted vagus nerve wellness routine can significantly enhance your overall health, reduce stress, and promote emotional resilience, creating a balanced life for years to come.

Conclusion

As you step into the transformative journey of nurturing and strengthening your vagus nerve, remember that every small action you take is a powerful investment in your health, well-being, and emotional resilience. The vagus nerve is not just a biological pathway; it is a bridge to your body's innate ability to heal, adapt, and thrive. Through intentional practices such as breathwork, mindfulness, movement, and cold exposure, you are actively participating in a process that will help you tap into your inner power, enhance your nervous system's balance, and elevate your life in ways you may have never imagined.

This journey is not a quick fix, but rather a lifelong commitment to yourself—one that requires patience, persistence, and self-compassion. By creating a personalized wellness routine centered around the vagus nerve, you are embracing the opportunity to transform your body's responses to stress, unlock deeper states of relaxation, and cultivate emotional balance that supports every aspect of your life. Every breath, every stretch, every act of kindness toward yourself, and every moment of stillness brings you closer to a life of greater harmony and vitality.

You are not just engaging in exercises or techniques; you are reconnecting with your body's natural rhythm and rediscovering the profound connection between mind, body, and spirit. With every step you take, you empower yourself to reclaim your health, your peace, and your resilience in a world that constantly demands more.

As you move forward, trust in your ability to create lasting change. Let this book serve as your guide, but always remember—the true power lies within you. You are the architect of your health, and through conscious, intentional practices, you have the ability to shape a future that is calm, balanced, and vibrant.

Your vagus nerve is a gateway to profound well-being, and now, you hold the key to unlock its full potential. Embrace this journey with confidence, knowing that the path you walk leads to a life of greater fulfillment, vitality, and peace.

The choice is yours. Step forward with intention, and let the transformation begin.

Bonus

Self Affirmation

As you embark on the journey of vagus nerve stimulation and wellness, it's essential to recognize the power of your mindset. The path to lasting transformation requires not only physical effort but also a mental foundation grounded in perseverance, determination, and belief in your own abilities. Your thoughts shape your reality, and when paired with the exercises, techniques, and practices outlined in this book, a resilient and empowered mindset will be your greatest ally. With each step forward, you are becoming stronger, more focused, and more capable of facing challenges with grace and strength.

Affirmations are powerful tools that can help shift your perspective, rewire your brain for success, and align your intentions with your goals. These affirmations, rooted in the principles of vagus nerve health and personal empowerment, will remind you of your innate strength and resilience. Allow them to inspire and guide you as you continue this life-enhancing journey.

10 Powerful Affirmations for Perseverance and Determination:

1. I am in control of my mind, body, and spirit, and I trust in my ability to heal and thrive.

2. Every breath I take strengthens my connection to my inner power and enhances my resilience.

3. With each step I take, I grow stronger, more balanced, and more aligned with my highest potential.

4. I embrace challenges as opportunities for growth, knowing that I have the strength to overcome them.

5. I am committed to my well-being, and I honor my body by nourishing it with practices that support my health.

6. My vagus nerve is a gateway to my vitality, and I actively work to enhance its function each day.

7. I am patient with myself, understanding that transformation is a process that requires time, consistency, and love.

8. I choose to focus on what I can control, and I take positive, purposeful actions toward my health and wellness every day.

9. I trust in my body's natural ability to heal, and I support it with practices that nurture my nervous system and emotional well-being.

10. I am dedicated to creating a life of peace, balance, and vitality, and I remain steadfast in my commitment to my journey.

These affirmations are reminders that you have everything you need within you to create meaningful change. They are not just words—they are declarations of the strength, resilience, and determination you possess. Embrace them daily, and watch as your mindset shifts to match the powerful transformation you are creating in your life.

Made in the USA
Monee, IL
07 September 2025